Don't Let It Smoke You

Don't Let It Smoke You

How to Create a Nontoxic Relationship with Cannabis

Tarris Batiste

JONES MEDIA PUBLISHING

For the readers.
Weed can have power over you, whether you're
using it medically or recreationally—smoke it,
but don't let it smoke you.

Contents

Acknowledgements

I could never express how grateful I am for my family—as well as the people who had a hand in helping me create this book. Thank you for encouraging me throughout this experience.

Writing this book made me seek balance in all areas of my life. Without it, I couldn't have gotten to where I am today. Finding balance has served me well—and I hope I can help others seek balance within their lives.

Our world is a better place thanks to people who want to develop and help others. What makes it even better are those who share the gift of their time to help change the trajectory of thinking for our future leaders.

Thank you.

Introduction

One conversation, one choice, and one action can cause a ripple effect in someone's life.

A choice I made in seventh grade—to smoke weed for the first time—ended up altering my life and my friends' lives. Without realizing it, we each developed a habit that changed us. We went from having huge dreams and aspirations to not giving a shit about anything. I started using weed to avoid dealing with my emotions. Any problems I faced, I just rolled into blunts. Over time, I felt like I had no control over my habit. It's as if invisible strings were pulling me, making me want to smoke any chance I could get. I felt like a pawn in a game of chess. As someone who loves freedom, I knew I had to change. But I didn't actually think I had a problem with weed until I reached my twenties.

This book is a reflection of the choices I made from middle school through college, which resulted in many detours in my future. Once on the verge of playing football for the Atlanta Falcons, I switched paths from being an athlete to an advocate of entrepreneurship. After my football career was cut short, I knew I needed to figure out a new direction for myself. (I couldn't keep smoking my problems away.) I started questioning why I was having so much difficulty shaking my smoking habit. This led me to travel, interview people, and do research on the history of cannabis. Through this process I was educated on how cannabis affects the brain, the trend of legalization in society, and what this all means for our youth.

In this book, I share my struggles with smoking weed, how and why I formed a habit, how I used it to numb my feelings and avoid facing problems, and how I eventually gained control of my habit through self-awareness. I created a system that helped me achieve balance, while becoming more aware of my own patterns and triggers that drove me to smoke. I share that system in later chapters.

My hope is that this book will inspire you to reflect so that you can make positive changes in your own life. This book is for anyone who wants to gain control over their smoking habit (or any other habit that's harming their life). You can use my system and tailor it to your unique situation.

My relationship with weed has always been complicated. I've battled with smoking for a long time. If I've learned anything, it's that being a prisoner of weed is no way to live. I felt captive. I knew my habit was blocking me from reaching my full potential, so something had to change. But nothing would change until I gained the awareness of how to create balance.

This is my story.

Note on usage: Throughout this book, I use the terms weed, cannabis, and marijuana interchangeably. Although there are many different forms with varying psychoactive effects, I'm specifically referring to smoking weed throughout this book.

Weed *symbolically represents a younger version of me, where I was using more of a street-level drug. That's what we called it when we were younger.*

Marijuana *is what they called it more in the past, using the term to create negative stigma.*

Cannabis *is rolling out now. It's more the scientific, harmless-sounding term—what they call it when they legalize it in your state or county.*

CHAPTER 1:
THE SECOND TIME
I SMOKED

In the summer of 2006, I was about to enter the seventh grade. Leaving behind childish things, like tic-tac-toe and tag games , I was excited to start my second year of middle school. That summer, I wanted to be productive and transform myself. So, I worked on my stutter and my basketball skills. I was young and just wanted to be seen. Little did I know my innocence would soon be challenged at the age of twelve—by weed.

A month before the new school year started, I had the opportunity to watch the high-school basketball team practice. I observed them, trying to memorize all their moves. I showed up again and again at practices. One day, one of the older kids noticed me.

He approached me and said, "Yo, youngsta, what's your name?"

"TB," I answered. Conscious of my stutter, I wanted to keep it short.

"Okay, TB. My name's Wild. What position do you play?" he asked.

"Point guard."

"No shit. Me too," he said. "We'll have to connect after practice. Maybe I can give you a few tips to help your game."

"All right, cool," I said.

It was a big deal to be noticed by the high schoolers. They were pros in my eyes.

Meeting Wild was the start of a new beginning. I went from shooting ball with him and the others to doing anything and everything they did. As time went on, being around them led to improvements in my game, but I also picked up an unexpected habit along the way.

One day after practice, Wild and his crew invited me to play in a four-game basketball tournament. I was nervous to play, but eager to showcase my skills on the court. During the first game, nothing was lining up for me. I aimed to play quality defense. I intended to break away and score a layup. As we went into the second half, my stats read 0 across the board. This inspired me to play harder. I desperately wanted to be valued in my team's eyes.

We won the game, but I was gravely disappointed in my inability to perform. It wasn't until game three that I started making strides. By this game, I had made four shots and was doing my best to be consistent. In the final minute, I stole the ball from the opposing team. I sprinted down the court for one more shot. I hesitated—instead of shooting, I passed the ball to Wild. He leapt through the air and dunked the basketball. We won the game and the tournament.

The team burst into a cheer. They embraced me in celebration.

Later that night, we celebrated at Cici's Pizza in Cartersville, Georgia. The guys joked, laughed, and told stories about the game. My teammates praised me. One of the players was eating everything in sight—I was like, "Damn, bro." At the time, I didn't know he was eating everything because he had smoked before the game and was high.

After we finished our dinner, Wild and his friends offered to drive me home. On the way back to my house, he asked me if I smoked. I paused and said, "Yeah, I mean, I could." He reached into the glove compartment and pulled out a few joints. He sparked one and began smoking. It seemed like this was second nature to him and his friends.

I was frightened at the possibility of getting caught by the police. Play, who was in the passenger seat, reached to pass me the joint. I hesitated, with conflicting thoughts going through my head, *Am I being a follower? Or am I not? Should I do it? Or should I not?* Growing up, my dad had always taught me not to be a follower. I wanted to make decisions based on what I thought, not what somebody else told me to do.

I reached forward to grab the joint anyway. I thought I was proving myself to be cool enough to hang with the older kids. I had no idea what I was doing or what I was signing up for. I learned about smoking from films or watching people do it in public. I smoked but wasn't sure if I inhaled it right, because I didn't feel any different right away.

Truthfully. I didn't fully understand the psychoactive effects cannabis had until the second time I smoked with Wild. I wasn't prepared for the odd sensation that hit me. The music in the background seemed to amplify, as if someone plugged the radio system into my brain and cranked up the volume. I felt a combination of clarity and relaxation. It was fun. I now had a taste of what smoking weed was to other people, and why they made such a big deal out of it. The hype that followed smoking proved itself to be true. I felt at ease and enjoyed the laughter and jokes that came along with it.

That's all it was at first—something that felt good and promoted laughter.

My Influence Reaching My Friends

I enjoyed smoking so much, I was excited to show it to my group of friends back at Cass Middle School.

I taught them how to roll up and smoke, just like Wild and his crew had taught me. From there, we all developed a deeper interest in smoking and different ways of doing it. We were young enthusiasts who wanted to experience everything weed had to offer.

By my eighth-grade year, my friends and I were smoking almost every day. We started seeing things through a different lens that made whatever was going on around us at any given moment less important. When we failed to execute in sports, or if we had a bad practice or game, the coach would bring us in for his after-the-game speech, with his veins popping out of his neck as he yelled at us. We'd look at each other with a smirk on our face like, "It's not that serious. We'll smoke this off tonight."

Even when things went well and we won, we celebrated by smoking. Slowly, some of my friends started showing up to first period high and giggly. I couldn't personally pull that off, because my parents wouldn't allow it. That's when our behavior began to shift.

As we got to high school, our smoking habit grew. It affected us in our own personal ways. My friend Q had been the best athlete and hardest worker out of all of us. He slowly disengaged from life. He threaded his whole life around smoking. He showed up high everywhere, every time, every minute, barely functioning. That was entirely unlike Q. He grew careless about all the things that were important to him before.

The scholar student out of us, Runt, was brilliant and blessed with brains, very smart in literature and English. We saw him drop out in the early years of high school, not giving a damn. He came into class one day with a pink slip for our teacher to sign. Although I had seen this coming, there was nothing I could say or do to stop him.

My friend Ant lost the battle way too soon. His personality changed the fastest. He went from being a people person to distancing himself from his friends and his family. He'd always been respectful, but once he started smoking, he began having this nonchalant, 'I couldn't care less' attitude.

Then there was me. Instead of handling my problems, I rolled them up and smoked them. I did that with everything, no matter what or who the problem was with—school, sports, family, or friends. If my friends and I argued, instead of talking it out, I'd say, "Who cares?" and go roll up. I smoked, and all my worries vanished—at least for the moment—but when I came down, I would just roll another one and get high again.

Truth be told, I used weed for recreation and medication. I never felt it was necessary to take pills (even before it was mainstream). But after smoking consistently , weed became my 'go-to,' my best friend. I smoked any chance I could get—as long as I had enough time to 'get right,' so my folks wouldn't know. My mom was helping teach at my high school, and my dad was a firearms training instructor at the time. He was working nine-to-five then; when he came home, he would head straight to the gym. I knew his pattern, and it was super easy to dodge when I was trying to get high. To avoid my mom, I would wait until she went to school, then I'd roll up in the backyard, being paranoid as hell that she might come back because she forgot something. For the most part, I got away with hiding it from my parents. My dad had no clue for the longest time, which I thought was funny because he had a law enforcement background. "He arrests people for stuff like this all the time, but he doesn't know his own son does it?" I thought.

On the other hand, my mom knew the whole time. My eyes would be red. My fingers would smell like weed. I was so young and inexperienced, I would 'hot box,' and then walk into the house, not thinking I smelled like weed. Shortly after noticing my mother's dark looks, I knew she caught on to what I was doing, I did everything to try to cover up the smell: wearing cologne, using eye drops, concentrating on washing my hands and scrubbing my fingernails.

Meanwhile, my friends and I forgot about all the aspirations we'd talked about before. I wondered why we were drifting so far away from where we said we wanted to be. We didn't talk about our goals anymore. We didn't intend to lose sight of what we wanted, but we did. I was confused, but I still wasn't affected enough by our experiences to make any changes in my life at that time.

The main thing that helped shape my opinion was that smoking didn't hinder my performance so I kept doing it. I convinced myself I was the exception, that I could do my best without having weed affect me. I still earned As and Bs at school and did well in football and basketball. I was still involved in the community. I was checking off all my set tasks throughout the day and never felt like I was doing anything wrong. And that was the dangerous part—I didn't know weed was holding me back. I was young and enjoying myself and never thought about how much *time* I was wasting going to meet the plug (waiting on him most of the time) and going to grab something to roll it in, then . . . I was engrossed in smoking and was headed down a dangerous path, not knowing the consequences of it.

I was living a double life. Out in public, you'd never know I smoked, because I never publicized it. If I did smoke before public functions, I would take the proper precautions so that nobody knew. The only people aware of it would be my friends who smoked with me.

I've always felt responsible and guilty for being the one to introduce my middle school friends to cannabis. I can't ever pay back what was lost or undo the toxic journey that I put my friends on— which all started with that choice I made in seventh grade. Our impressionable, young minds couldn't have predicted that our lives would change so much. If only we'd been given a disclosure statement of all the possible side effects or outcomes of smoking; it may have changed some of the decisions we made.

All I can do is pay it forward and help those who face the same situations I did, so that you can make a conscious decision about what to smoke or when to smoke—and whether you're smoking it or if it's smoking you.

CHAPTER 2:
THE WEED WAVE

Cannabis is perceived in many different ways. Society has seen a shift in the popularity of cannabis: I refer to this as the "weed wave." Overall, the weed wave is the progressive acceptance that cannabis is establishing in society. People are starting to see cannabis as acceptable, especially with legalization in certain states.

Historically, people have always viewed weed as the "delinquent child" in society, but now it's become extremely popular for its positive effects. We've seen substances like alcohol and tobacco increase in popularity, but time showed us their negative side effects.

Cannabis is now reaching its peak. There's a societal debate on how much people should use cannabis and what it should be used for. Is it good or bad for your body? How much of it can (or should) you consume? What's the impact? I predict cannabis will be legal everywhere within the next couple of years of this writing. Regardless of legalization, I've recognized several things about this substance.

From "Demonized" to "Highly Sought After"

In the past, many people demonized cannabis without understanding the nature of the plant. Medical technology has shown the pros and cons of cannabis, which I'll discuss later in this book. There is value in researching cannabis to understand its overall effects. What amount of consumption is classified as addiction? Experience has shown me that if cannabis is abused, it can highly disrupt your life. I've witnessed the struggle and severe influence cannabis has had on the lives of my family, friends, colleagues, and even myself.

Everybody has that one person in the family that takes a rougher path, often establishing habits in the next generation of family members. Whether those habits are good or bad, a majority of the time they're passed down. It's that person in your family that always teaches you not to make the same mistakes that they have, yet never seeks to change their own ways. I've seen multiple people in my family fear opportunities that could have changed their life and put them in an upward trajectory— and they let weed get in front of that. I didn't like the fact that some of my family members would cap themselves, that dreaming was merely a concept that had its own bounds. I didn't want to follow in that same path. I felt like I was becoming that "next person" in my family who did all of that. I knew I had to correct myself. Once I faced my dependency, I realized I wasn't alone. I connected with other people who had similar experiences and were on the same path of becoming aware of their dependency.

As I reflect on my life and the stories of others I spoke with, I wonder whether I would have been on the same path if cannabis was legalized in Georgia while I was growing up. I probably would've found myself in a much different scenario with all the discreet ways you can consume cannabis with its legalization.

Legalization is encouraging a new generation of people to have substance dependency. Why is that? I would say more than likely for the profit and business opportunity behind it. Legalization and decriminalization are beneficial for both the state and federal government. The state specifically benefits from cannabis being taxed. This lets the state be reimbursed for previous expenses, due to conviction and care for charged individuals. (Later in the book I discuss the history of cannabis to present day.) This highlights the expenses and resources needed to fund those who are incarcerated. They can generate money from taxes to fund the state's needs and essentially cut the corrections budget. Not only does it affect the population's health, but also people's income.

Cannabis shops are set up in lower-class communities, which contribute to another socioeconomic problem. Although many people of various economic backgrounds use cannabis, it's interesting how a shop is more often placed in a low-income area than in an area with a higher-income bracket. For example, in the area I live in, several shops surround me. But when I'm in a well-developed neighborhood, dispensaries seem to be placed out of sight, out of mind. According to the *Marijuana Business Daily*, 40 percent of cannabis shops in Seattle and approximately 45 percent in Denver are placed in areas where average income is in the bottom 25th percentile.[1] Regardless of dispensaries being strategically placed in these areas, the dependency that comes with cannabis doesn't discriminate against economic status. It will get you whether you're rich or poor.

Being a collegiate athlete and briefly playing for the Atlanta Falcons, I saw how cannabis impacted both college students and athletes. Transitioning out of my redshirt season I remember idolizing Tyrann Mathieu who played for LSU. He was one of the best cornerbacks in college football and was a Heisman candidate.

I remember the day I was watching the announcement of his dismissal from LSU due to multiple failed drug tests. I was surprised with the fact that a high nationally ranked athlete struggled to discipline himself in order to keep his scholarship. How could someone with so much potential find himself in such a predicament?

Then I would hear about Johnny Manziel and Josh Gordon on ESPN, who were both high-level football players that struggled with smoking. Johnny Manziel wasn't as fortunate, and his career slowly faded after several reoccurring incidents. While playing in the NFL, Josh Gordon ended up getting suspended multiple times before finding a spot with the Seattle Seahawks.

As time went on, the media revealed several athletes that struggled with smoking weed. All these professionals were still relatable, because they too had to work just as hard to discipline themselves. The only difference I see is that the average person doesn't have the same resources as professional athletes. What happens to the average person with the same struggle?

Tyrann Mathieu and Josh Gordon are potential assets that had the resources to help them. Their position gave them the opportunity to get treatment in order to get them back to playing as soon as possible. However, the average person doesn't have the same foothold, and more don't than do. So how are others like me able to help themselves without the same resources or care?

When I played football at Georgia State, only about twenty out of almost one hundred players on the team didn't smoke. Many of us got into a routine of smoking consistently throughout college, but it didn't stop there. I saw teammates' smoking habits follow them after college football. Little did I know, I would also see this trend in my short-lived experience attending a rookie minicamp in the NFL.

Based on the number of NFL players who smoke and are allowed to do so, I predict professional athletes will have cannabis sponsorships and partnerships in the future. This will have a huge impact on aspiring athletes' lifestyles. If you grow up watching your favorite players endorse, smoke, or support cannabis, it can make the drug seem harmless.

Think of it this way: Michael Jordan is an iconic basketball player with his own brand. He partnered with Nike, which helped elevate his brand. Soon everyone became obsessed with the merchandise he endorsed, from Air Jordan to his vintage apparel line. People who may not have even watched basketball watched him and bought his merchandise. Now, if we change Michael Jordan's shoe to a cannabis endorsement, what's the result? Does it change the way kids view cannabis?

Even though it may seem harmless, it's hard to say the younger generation will understand cannabis for all it is. It's easy to assume it's okay to consume cannabis if it's legal and if professional athletes do it. As much as the professional athlete has fame and influence, the general youth doesn't have their same set of circumstances, nor can they apply those same actions to their personal life. The youth are still in the process of growing and learning discipline and balance in their own life.

A Susceptible Generation

Society has glamorized this drug with billboards, celebrities, and social media ads. We've gotten to the point where professional athletes and celebrities have publicly come out about their personal use or cannabis business. LeBron James's son was caught smoking weed on his Instagram. Barack Obama's daughter was also caught several years ago smoking at a concert. This is the new normal. It would be silly to say that these popular figures don't have some type of influence on our youth. Not to mention the NFL and NBA have just relaxed their policies on cannabis usage.

What is the legalization of cannabis all about, and what's behind it? This industry targets young kids and gets them hooked to becoming lifelong customers. At a young age, I was influenced without knowing the effects. I had limited awareness and made impulsive decisions that weren't suited for long-term success. I realize cannabis isn't the worst thing out there, but that's why it can be so dangerous—you justify it because it's "harmless" or "not that bad." It's one of those drugs that's easy to abuse and that can become an issue before you know it.

Studies show that during adolescence and prior to brain maturity at age twenty-five, cannabis causes structural damage to the brain, which can lead to a lifetime of addiction. Many of my young friends and family members love to get high, and I've been with each one of them at some point during smoke sessions. In a way, the decision to smoke binds people together. This leads to long-term cultural change.

Without having the initiative to change, sometimes we can trap ourselves in a never-ending cycle where all we do is look to get high throughout the day. We go through each day using cannabis as a synthetic burst of happiness or relaxation. Knowledge can help young people at least have a chance to change. I want all youth to have the ability to change their lives and create a legacy that moves forward. With legalization approaching all fifty states, young minds need education. I can't make younger people listen—hell, I hardly listened and still don't most of the time—all I can do is reveal the truth and hope people will choose their potential and legacy over getting high.

Proceed with Caution

If you bring cannabis into your daily life in an unhealthy way, you'll start to need it more than you enjoy it. I don't want to convince you to stop using cannabis, but rather to practice discipline around your usage of it (if you choose to use it at all). The reason cannabis becomes a drug is because people let it become one. You might go through a phase where you feel like you depend on getting high to enjoy your day. That was me for years; I couldn't stand the feeling of being out of control and going through the motions knowing damn well I should've been saving the extra cash I had. If you don't find balance and act disciplined, the substance can harm you. The popular saying, "Too much of anything is bad for you," is true. We live in a time where many things that don't have to be bad for us have become drugs, like food, coffee, alcohol, and technology. You can enjoy all of these things occasionally, but if you overuse them, they become harmful to your mind and body

I hope you'll proceed with caution. I was someone who felt consumed by cannabis and had no control. What shaped my opinion is the research I did and the questions I asked. I immersed myself in the controversy surrounding cannabis and then came to my own conclusions.

Chapter 2 Summary

1. The weed wave has slowly become popular and marketed, after being demonized in the past.

2. Ask yourself: Is cannabis limiting you, and to what extent?

3. Our world has become more centralized around social media and has proven to be paving its way with future generations. With legalization, cannabis has the ability to weave its way into several different avenues that could impact the youth.

4. Be sure to do your research and educate yourself on the downsides of smoking weed. Without having a full understanding, you can easily let something control you.

CHAPTER 3:
A GREEN HISTORY

Coming into my midtwenties, I became curious about the history of cannabis and its popularity within my generation. I was interested in how people of all cultures used cannabis and why it was restricted in the United States. Originally, I wanted to prove to myself that cannabis wasn't as bad as people framed it to be. This led me to a series of questions related to the events leading up to legalization.

As I researched cannabis, new findings gave me a better understanding. Cannabis has been around for longer than most people think. Digging into the origin of the plant, I saw how different cultures viewed cannabis and how this set the stage for legalization.

Our Stigmatized Past

Cannabis has been around since the BC era. It's been called different names and has been used in many regions across the world in different ways. Dating back to the ancient civilizations in Asia Minor, China, Europe, and the Middle East, cannabis was used for medicinal, recreational, and spiritual purposes. In the Middle East, people referred to cannabis as *hashish*. Hashish was mainly smoked and used for spiritual rituals.

In ancient China, cannabis was known as the hemp seed flower, or *hemp*. China was one of the first cultivators of cannabis and mainly used it for clothing, rope, medicine, and cooking. Cannabis was a vital crop because it could easily be grown anywhere, which made it great for farming. The fibers were versatile and were used to make everything at that time.

Cannabis made its way to North America in the mid-1700s and slowly spread to other parts of the world. Cannabis became a common ingredient used in different medicines. It was most known to be used in tinctures. Tinctures were liquid concentrates created by mixing the plant with alcohol to pull out active ingredients. Through the 1800s, marijuana remained harmless and was experimented with in medicine.[2]

During the 1900s, people started to question the effects of cannabis and whether it should be used solely for medicinal purposes, or for recreational use and entertainment. The United States found reasons that ruled cannabis as harmful and problematic. The properties cannabis was known for in the past slowly shifted from medicinal to recreational.

During the Mexican revolutionary era, people changed their perception of marijuana. Instead of using it medically, people began smoking it recreationally. From 1910 to 1920, over 100,000 Mexicans immigrated into the United States. They brought with them a new form of consumption to the citizens of America. Prior history never projected the recreational use of marijuana, striking a red flag. People noticed how Mexicans used the plant and began to copy this. Soon, smoking the plant entered the American consciousness and became popular.

In 1913, California created a bill criminalizing cannabis. Pushed by the Board of Pharmacy, the bill served as a way to regulate opiates and psychoactive pharmaceuticals. As laws were pushed by special interest groups rather than actual doctors, critics raised questions about marijuana. That paved the way to a full ban in the 1930s.

Society Gets Programmed

In 1930, the Federal Bureau of Narcotics was introduced, and Harry Anslinger was the first director. He was one of the primary people responsible for fabricating the stigma around cannabis. As director, he launched a campaign against cannabis that would hold steady for decades. Anslinger continued shaping the negative image of cannabis and pushed to change the name of the drug to *marijuana*, which is what Mexican people called it in their culture. Anslinger knew if he kept programming the word *marijuana* into people's brains, that word would get entangled with the Mexican immigrants.[3]

Anslinger used creative avenues to convey his message. He provided movie theaters with commercials that racialized cannabis, making white audiences despise the drug. Anslinger went to Congress explaining that "marijuana is the most violence-causing drug in the history of mankind. . . . Most marijuana smokers are Negroes, Hispanics, Filipinos and entertainers. Their satanic music, jazz and swing, result from marijuana usage." Anslinger also reported, "Reefer makes darkies think they're as good as white men."[4] Anslinger did everything possible to slander the image of minorities by orchestrating films like *Reefer Madness* and *The Devil's Lettuce*. These films were intended to influence others into thinking people who used marijuana were evil and killers. He was successful at selling his perspective, as many Americans shared this same outlook.

Anslinger wrote the Marijuana Tax Act of 1937, which federally criminalized cannabis in every U.S. state. The Tax Act placed a one-dollar tax on anyone who sold or cultivated cannabis. Individuals also had to comply with certain enforcement provisions.

Any violation of the provisions would result in imprisonment or a fine of up to $2,000, roughly equivalent to $35,500 today, or both.

The United States slowly created a wave of doubt about the true effects of marijuana, which led to further penalties in the future. Disagreements and opposition came from citizens against criminalization. This created conflict and restrictions to completely rule out the use of marijuana. The Boggs Act of 1951 made mandatory jail sentences for all people using cannabis. To limit offenses of usage, the Narcotics Control Act of 1956 was introduced to provide worse consequences.

In 1970, before Nixon stepped into office, the federal government passed the Controlled Substance Act (CSA). Soon after, Nixon started the "war on drugs" in the 1970s during his administration. In 1971, during a press conference, he called drug abuse the "public enemy number one problem." Two years later, in 1973, he created the Drug Enforcement Administration (DEA) to enforce those federal drug laws.

That same year, the state of Oregon decriminalized the drug. Oregon did this because of the Preemption Clause found in the CSA. The

Preemption Clause allows states to legalize cannabis if they want to. Normally, federal law wins over state laws, but because of the Preemption Clause, the federal laws can't override all state drug laws. The clause is how Oregon decriminalized cannabis contrary to every other state at the time.

The downside was that enforcing laws against cannabis was costing states millions of dollars. This realization sparked California to create a new set of laws in 1976 that reduced the penalty for possession of less than an ounce of marijuana. The penalty was no longer a felony and would be considered a misdemeanor with a maximum fine.

Going into the 1980s, the Reagan administration reinstated the Anti-Drug Abuse Act in 1986. The Act was related to the distribution of cannabis, and with a future amendment, it added a twenty-five-year imprisonment for crimes committed three times. By that time, the Reagan's "Just Say No" campaign arrived. The war on drugs was in full swing. They tried to find new ways to commercialize and advertise how harmful drugs were. If you're old enough, you may remember the D.A.R.E program (Drug Abuse Resistance Education). It was introduced to steer adolescents away from using drugs. It was a program meant to help children become educated and choose to be drug free, but some critics think it increased drug usage among youth.

While Anslinger, Nixon, and Reagan were in office, many people were locked up, and they feared drug-related punishments. The severity of using or possessing marijuana was progressively getting worse. In the 1990s, the incarceration rates in the United States vastly increased. The United States had the highest incarceration rates in the world at the time, with a majority being minorities.

Approaching Present Day

In 1996, things started to shift, and California passed Proposition 215, which legalized cannabis. California helped shift the ideas of cannabis, and other states soon began to follow. Colorado and Washington would be next, legalizing adult use in 2012. Positive attention was generated around the economic value within these states that soon led to the legalization movement.

Now nearing the end of 2020, we have roughly eleven states fully legalized, twenty-one with medical legalization, and a few states are decriminalized without legalization. Hopefully, as cannabis becomes more acceptable, more states will decriminalize the drug as well. People will be able to buy cannabis in a more controlled environment rather than just off the streets.

After understanding the history and gaining insight on both perspectives, it seems that cannabis is used as a means to an end for specific agendas. The foundation of making cannabis illegal was to incarcerate and deport minorities. I often wondered why cannabis was suddenly becoming legalized and more mainstream. Now it's in their favor to legalize cannabis for business opportunities and profit.

I believe we'll start to see legalization spread to all fifty states in some form or fashion. The amount of money used in the past to control the substance has proven itself to be senseless. If the United States legalizes cannabis throughout the entire country, I expect there will be many adjustments and decisions to be made in terms of convictions or felonies for possession or selling. It will be interesting to see how enforcements of the past will change to align with the overall legalization movement.

Chapter 3 Summary

1. Cannabis has been around since the BC era; however the uses were normally medicinal. The Mexican revolutionary era was when recreational marijuana became popular and crossed over into the United States.

2. Anslinger used his position and avenues to racialize cannabis and tied it to minorities. He also advertised the negatives of the drug and enforced programs and laws that supported his view.

3. Society seemed to be programmed into believing that cannabis was a very negative drug that was highly addictive, outweighing the benefits.

4. In the end California pressed forward to legalize cannabis in 1996; Colorado, Oregon, and Washington followed shortly after. Now in 2020 we have seen more states legalize and decriminalize marijuana, and I predict it won't be long before it's legalized everywhere.

CHAPTER 4:
THE SEARCH

In my pursuit to understand cannabis, I did research online. I wasn't satisfied with what I was reading, so in 2018, while I was getting my master's degree at Georgia State University, I had a vision to seek out three people who had knowledge of the cannabis industry. I saved up money for any travel expenses: I valeted at night, woke up at five a.m. to be a full-time graduate assistant, then after work, headed to my five-hour class. That was my routine. After six months, I had enough money saved up to see my project through.

I wanted to interview three people who could make my research valuable and sensible. I decided to connect with one person who was pro cannabis, one who was against it, and one who could shed light on what happens to the brain after short- or long-term use of cannabis. Anyone else I spoke with along the way would be a bonus to my research. I searched for people and companies whom I felt met my qualifications. I emailed over fifty people a day for two months just to see who I could get to sit down with me. I got on the phone with some pretty cool people who gave me tons of great feedback about the legalization and innovation around cannabis. I finally found my "big three" individuals whom I could take a trip to speak with.

Kevin Damata on the Economic Benefits of Legalizing Cannabis

My first stop was Denver, Colorado, in November 2018. I met with Kevin Damata, the social media manager and video producer for the Adagio Bud and Breakfast Hotel. He took me through his positive views on cannabis. In Denver,

Colorado, mass legalization of cannabis has led to normal use of the drug and innovative businesses.

At the Bud and Breakfast, I met up with Damata, and he shed light on cannabis from a business standpoint. The Bud and Breakfast opened in 2016. This unique hotel experience has been fully booked just by being one of the first to offer a cannabis-friendly stay. The hospitality was great for cannabis enthusiasts and showed how cannabis has been beneficial to business.

Waiting to speak with Damata, I ran into some of the guests staying at the Adagio. After informing them why I was there, they kindly gave me their personal reviews on the hotel. They spoke of their favorite strains and showed me unique bongs and other creative smoking pieces available at the hotel. From what they told me, I think that the Bud and Breakfast meets the needs of the specific audience they're trying to attract.

Shortly after my personal tour I got to talk to Damata and interviewed him about his thoughts on the weed wave. From speaking with him I was able to gain clarity on some of the good things about legalization. The one thing he favored about cannabis was that it is more natural compared to other drugs out there. This is something I could relate to, because as a football player I preferred cannabis rather than pharmaceuticals for pain. Cannabis might be addictive, but in its natural state it won't lead to overdose or fatality.

I learned that the human body has an endocannabinoid system, which works to keep your body balanced after experiencing stress, pain, inflammation, and more. Our body naturally produces similar compounds that are found in cannabis.

Damata believes there's value in using cannabis-derived products versus other unnatural products. He specifically pointed out the history of Coca-Cola and it ironically being named after the coca leaf (the same ingredient used to make cocaine). Coca-Cola no longer uses the coca leaf as the source of caffiene in the drinks, but the fact is that the ingredients used aren't all that healthy anyways. For this reason Damata believes that cannabis industries have an opportunity to create similar products in a more natural way than its competition.

Could companies like Coca-Cola take a backseat to cannabis companies? Cannabis has definitely been seen in different products that have been found useful. Damata thinks that bigger companies and pharmaceutical companies fell behind, while cannabis has progressively been making its way into different markets. Now there's Canna Cola and CBD oils and creams that have been found helpful with reducing inflammation and increasing focus. Those companies don't want the drug legalized until they've caught up. Damata emphasized how cannabis makers have had nothing but time to perfect different products that are transparent and better than the competition.

The cannabis industry has had a profitable impact on the economy and has helped develop the area and nearby communities in Denver. The taxes from legalization could potentially change the economic scope of many states. The major perks of the booming cannabis industry are that it can create more businesses. This is seen in areas where legalization has taken place. There's no doubt the industry has a large following. It provides jobs for both production and business aspects, which leads to a wide range of occupations. Shops have gone up everywhere and places similar to the Adagio Bud and Breakfast create an attractive experience to those who desire to smoke freely.

Damata talked about the surrounding area being full of run-down homes and empty factories. Those homes and factories were renovated and became grow houses and cannabis-friendly yoga studios to promote the overall experience. Damata spoke highly of the changes that have been made in the Denver community, resulting in a more profitable state.

Carla Lowe and Roger Morgan on the Downfalls of Cannabis Legalization

My second stop was to Sacramento, California, in November 2018, to meet Carla Lowe (the Founder of Citizens Against Marijuana) and Roger Morgan (founder of the Take Back America Campaign) to discuss concerns about continued legalization. Here is a little background on Carla Lowe: she organized one of the nation's first "parent/community" groups in Sacramento, cofounded Californians for Drug-Free Youth, chaired the Nancy Reagan Speakers' Bureau of the National Federation of Parents for Drug-Free Youth, cofounded Californians for Drug-Free

Schools, and in 2010 founded Citizens Against Legalizing Marijuana (CALM).

I learned Lowe's perspective of the cannabis industry. I was intrigued by her background and wanted to know why she was fighting so hard to warn people about legalization. Lowe has traveled over 400,000 miles in the U.S. and around the world speaking about marijuana's impact on young people and society. In 2014, she helped organize, and served as president of Americans Against Legalizing Marijuana, a nonprofit organization that educates lawyers by providing legal and scientific guidance so that they can take the marijuana industry to court.

Being able to speak with Lowe was amazing, and I greatly appreciated the time she spent conversing with me. From the beginning I noticed the extra effort she put into educating me. I arrived finding out that she invited Roger Morgan, the founder of the Take Back America campaign.

Lowe and Morgan gave me additional information from brochures, including the negative aspects of cannabis. We had a dialogue, and exchanged our views about the future of cannabis. I talked about the impact that I've seen within the

Black community. I also explained what I wrote in reference to the weed wave. They were shocked by some of the points I mentioned, because it never crossed their mind. I explained how smoking was associated with the Black culture, and how it's often used as an aid. To further describe my perspective, I pointed out how rap music tends to normalize smoking. Then you have big entertainers like Dave Chappell that star in movies where smoking is framed as if it's accepted. Typically, this is something that is personified within the black community.

After expressing concerns of cannabis, we both noticed that the media has played a major role in pushing overall acceptance. The conversation added value to my learning process, and I found that some of our beliefs were aligned.

Out of the information they mentioned, I found a few interesting points that stuck out to me. One of the first points Lowe mentioned is how cannabis is a fat-soluble, mind-altering, highly toxic drug that remains in the body and brain for a minimum of one month, building up with each additional use. Lowe and Morgan mentioned emotional maturity being delayed for young users. As young minds are growing, they're learning to adapt and cope with social, emotional, and physical stressors. When cannabis is introduced at a young age, it disrupts this process. In adolescence, it's important to allow proper development of the brain, and cannabis can prolong that process. Cannabis can be a buffer for high stress and overall interfere with learning to cope in a healthy way. I would agree with this information, given that I've struggled firsthand with learning healthy ways to cope with my stressors.

Lowe also touched on the change in THC (tetrahydrocannabinol) levels that was alarming. The potency of THC within cannabis used to be 2 percent and today it has increased to over 20 percent. This can heavily impact brain development.

Also, for all my earth-conscious people, I learned how the production of cannabis causes irreparable damage to the ecosystem by damaging natural resources. Morgan informed me that one marijuana plant can consume up to six gallons of water per day. This diverts water from streams, creating issues for wildlife habitats. Also, with pesticides being used for cultivation, the runoff can impact wildlife negatively.

This information gave me a greater understanding about some of the main concern's legalization can bring. Next, I was ready to learn about the side effects of cannabis, as explained by science and medicine.

Dr. Michael Kuhar on How Cannabis Disrupts Brain Function and Development

My last resource was Michael Kuhar, author of *The Addicted Brain* and neuroscientist at Emory University in Atlanta, Georgia. Dr. Kuhar taught me how cannabis works with natural processes in the body and how it disrupts brain function. He articulated the scientific process that Carla Lowe and Roger Morgan had referred to.

Dr. Kuhar explained his views of short-term and long-term memory and how they're affected by cannabis. He strongly believes you're at risk of losing a major part of your long-term memory, even if you only consume once a week. Also, the earlier you start using cannabis, the more it impacts your IQ development. If you smoke consistently you might struggle with being able to access your experiences and what you've learned throughout the years. Dr. Kuhar considers cannabis will be a challenge in the future for some, not for all. The momentum of the medical movement and the recreational movement suggest cannabis is not a very big problem. He feels society won't be able to fully understand how many people struggle with this drug, because there hasn't been enough data to pull from.

Dr. Kuhar began by explaining how drugs work in the brain by acting at receptors, which are small molecular sites that receive signals from neurons. Neurons are nerve cells that work in your body to sense and carry out an action. The neurons in our brain are used to communicate and pass information to these receptor sites. The receptors in our brain have naturally occurring processes that activate signals for us to do or feel certain things. Drugs that are abused interact with these systems but have a stronger effect. That effect is what makes you feel euphoric or relaxed. He described the receptors in the brain as a "switch" and the drug as a "finger." Whenever the finger hits the switch, a reaction takes place.

Dr. Kuhar's concern is that legalizing cannabis would be making it more psychologically available to kids. Young brains grow so rapidly, and nowadays with THC being so potent, it can cause serious dependency problems and disrupt brain development. Dr. Kuhar also referred to the lack of data on the amount of people who abuse cannabis. He explained:

> The current data demonstrates that 9 percent of heavy users become addicts. Although that doesn't sound like a lot, it's a huge number when you're talking about a serious problem. Think of it this way—would you go to the grocery store and buy food that has quality control issues 9 percent of the time? That means approximately one out of every ten times food would be bad. So, the level and the frequency of problems are big enough that people should pay attention and be aware of them.

Think about this when you hear about states passing a cannabis law. Do they give you any precautions or do they give you problems? One thing I would like you to consider is that not all cannabis is tested for purity and quality. There are plenty of cases online where cannabis has been found with mold, pesticide, or contamination or laced with other substances that are unhealthy for you.

People need to consider the company they purchase cannabis from, just as people are selective in buying produce from grocery stores. Because the FDA knows that cannabis is cultivated in ways that don't align with the public health, just recently in 2019 the FDA has begun to regulate cannabis and cannabis-derived products. Right now, you don't know what you're getting when purchasing cannabis from a legal retailer, and this will have an effect on your body in the long run. That's why in the near future people will probably grow their own food and grow their own weed—that's the only way to truly know if it's organic.

Let's take Whole Foods for example: they are a grocery store that specifically sells organically grown produce. Although it costs a little more, why not pay for your health now so that you don't have to pay later. Right? The only issue is that later people found out that the FDA's standards and regulations for what's considered organic was quite lenient. Turns out FDA organic doesn't technically mean you're getting 100 percent organic products. The lack of transparency led to third-party organizations testing for quality and abiding by proper standards of what can be classified as organic.

That's why it's important to do your research and find out what you're putting in your body, because the reality is that not all cannabis is good. There's cannabis that's grown more with a thought of money behind it than with the thought of tastefulness, or righteousness of how it's grown. You have to nurture the plant in certain ways as it grows—making sure it's in a healthy environment— and not just spraying it with whatever will increase production and potency. It's about quality control, not just genetically modifying the plant to make it grow faster.

I knew I had some checking and rethinking to do about cannabis. Dr. Kuhar gave me solid information that I believe everyone should know. Understanding all perspectives is vital to making the best possible decision before getting into something. I didn't do it to persuade or prove a point, I just wanted to have the facts, just as I believe everyone should. Learning what I did reminded me why it's so important to understand how cannabis can affect you. I had an issue and receiving the information that I did gave me a reason to gain total control over my smoking habit. At the end of the day, it's about being able to better yourself.

The way I used weed at that time had to change. Check yourself and make sure you're in control—and if you're not, it's about taking small steps to get there.

Chapter 4 Summary

1. Although cannabis has had negative views, the business side of the industry seems to bring value to the economy with providing several different jobs and attractions for tourism.

2. Cannabis also seems to be able to be a more natural way to produce different types of medicine or anti-inflammatories versus pharmaceuticals.

3. Cannabis being used at a young age has a negative impact on adolescent minds and bodies. This can disrupt development and set emotional maturity backwards.

4. THC levels used to be 2 percent and now they have increased to over 20 percent which has a harder impact on brain development— and the percentage will continue to increase overtime.

CHAPTER 5:
WEEDING IT OUT

To navigate my complicated relationship with weed, I sought direction and counsel in many places. One Sunday, while attending a sermon, I heard my pastor say, "The same thing you struggle with will be the same thing you use to bless others."

I've never heard a statement so true. I often struggled when learning to adapt to different lifestyle changes. I failed more times than I expected, and the knowledge I received from others made me want to analyze myself. Smoking affected my health, finances, mentality, relationships, and career. These areas suffered from misplaced focus and lack of awareness. The most important thing for me was to live out my values, not just state them. Reflecting and analyzing my struggles and failures gave me a different perspective on how to go about changing.

I refer to the initial changes as "weeding it out." Weeding it out is like the starting point of a thorough detox. I spent years trying to change my smoking patterns and failing. I went through every emotion trying to find something that worked best for my long-term success. After many failed attempts, and making many adjustments, I found my own personal solution to creating a strong foundation for constant change and improvement. I focused on three things: becoming conscious of my issues, creating balance within my patterns, and learning to consistently keep up with my values.

These three things build a strong foundation when you're making major changes. They're similar and as important as building a strong foundation for a house. Most people aren't aware that the foundation takes the most time to construct. It's the part that holds the entire weight of the house. Any cracks or weakness will result in structural damage to the house above ground. With a properly built foundation, a house will have less complications. We start by building our personal foundation so that we can make sustainable changes.

Acknowledge and Be Conscious of Your Issue

Acknowledging your smoking issue is the first step in changing it. This is what it means to be conscious of your issue. I once heard a successful business owner talking about change. He said, "In order for you to know where you're going, you have to know where you are." Look at it this way: if, for example, you're trying to get somewhere on a trail or hike, the first thing you look for is the placard with the red star that tells you where you are. Once you know where you are, you can see where and in what direction you need to go. Being aware of where you are gives you direction. Without it, you can end up somewhere unknown. That's how I look at acknowledgement—without it, you can't know where you're going if you aren't willing to admit you have an issue.

It took me years to acknowledge my issue with weed. The thought crossed my mind that I had a problem, but I was always reluctant to admit it. I didn't face my issue until I was in college, and even then, it wasn't my own doing. It was a comment my dealer made to me.

I remember the story like it was yesterday. During winter, I walked from campus to 625, which was a well-known football party house at Indiana State. Being from Georgia, I wasn't properly equipped to walk in the harsh winter of Terre Haute. I only had my football letterman's jacket to keep me warm. I walked two miles or more in the dead of winter just to get over an ounce of weed. As I arrived, my dealer opened the door. He greeted me and invited me in, peaking over my shoulder out the front door. Noticing no car out front, he asked, "Did you walk here from campus?"

"Yeah," I replied.

He laughed hysterically as he bagged the weed up and gave it to me. Now I know he was laughing at me walking in the conditions I did, for weed.

We made our way toward the stairway, leading to the foyer. Making our way to the front door, I reached for the doorknob. Before I could turn it, he firmly put his hand on my shoulder and said, "TB, make sure you don't let that shit smoke you."

I looked at him and nonchalantly nodded in agreement and walked out. When I tell that story out loud or even think about it, I feel crazy. I should've noticed the issue myself. The power of his words didn't set in until after that night. His comment confirmed an issue I hadn't been ready to admit. It was my "aha" moment. What I valued the most in life came second to smoking. Weed was a roadblock to me making the best choices for myself. That moment made me look at my life differently. I wanted to change how I thought about myself.

How do you acknowledge something you can't see? Sometimes another person has to expose your problem to you so that you can acknowledge you have an issue. The best and quickest way to find out if you lack control is to ask for an outside perspective. If you don't acknowledge your issue with smoking, it will waste more of your time. Time is precious, and it's something I wasted so much of, because I went through the first quarter of my life never asking about my own weaknesses. If I was intentional and asked those around me, I could have worked on changing sooner. That's why it's best to question your actions and always try to grow and do better. The alternative is waiting for life to show you, and that date shouldn't be unpredictable.

Becoming conscious of your issues and changing them can take time. There's a moment when people can accept the information and make physical changes. Experience has taught me that growth in certain areas or issues can't have a time limit. Most people told me things about smoking, and I didn't really hear what they were saying, but eventually I did.

Learn from my situation so that you can get a head start. Ask yourself and others close to you if they think you might have an issue with cannabis. That way, you can begin to grow.

Don't think that acknowledging your issue means you have to solve everything right away either. I wanted to quit so fast so that I could move forward. But that wasn't helpful for me. I felt frustrated, thinking I had to make drastic changes overnight. I was ready to quit before I started. Acknowledging your smoking problem is the first step. All it means is, you need to grow in that particular area. Value the small wins. It's a lifestyle change, so focus on becoming disciplined and stronger.

Balance: Finding Your Middle

At this point, it's not about quitting—it's about finding balance within your normal smoking patterns. This means finding your median or middle ground. This will be different for everyone, depending on what balance means to you. Balance can be recognized in two ways: The first is viewed from action or production. The second is viewed more as quantitative. For example, I think of balance in terms of production—what am I doing or producing each day? My desire to produce and succeed in areas I'm building has to come first, before smoking. If I wanted to smoke, it had to be *after* I checked off tasks I thought were valuable to my growth for that day. That was all it took for me to find my middle ground.

I have a brother who looks at balance from more of a quantitative perspective. Let's say he smoked four times a day and wanted to find his middle ground. A good balance for him would be to only smoke twice a day instead of four times—cutting back to half of what he's used to smoking. That would be a win.

These are both examples of balance. Depending on how you view balance, you might use one or both of these approaches to find your median. Finding that middle ground is an important step, so you're not over- or under-challenging yourself. It's similar to a seesaw or teeter-totter: one side is your smoking pattern, the other side is productivity. All I want is for you to balance your current smoking patterns the best you can. That means transferring some weight over to productivity. I want you to shift slightly. The goal is for you to be accustomed to your middle ground. Eventually it will become your new standard.

After I consistently accomplished balance within my daily routine, I only smoked twice a day. That may seem like a lot, but you're essentially cutting your normal pattern in half. Your 50 percent better than you were when you started. That's a great starting point and foundation to build on.

Maintaining Your Garden

Once you consistently keep up with your new standard, you'll gain confidence in your ability to grow beyond that. Consistency in this step is necessary for sustainable growth. Think of yourself as a garden. A garden produces whatever is planted. In order for that "produce" to continue growing, certain actions need to happen. A garden needs water, sunlight, fertile soil, and continuous maintenance. The maintenance also consists of defending your garden by removing any weeds that present themselves. If you don't pick the weeds, your garden will get overloaded and eventually it won't produce anything of value. The weeds will take over, and no matter how much you nurture your garden, it won't have room to grow. You must consistently keep weeds from stunting the shift you've made.

Advancing my own garden took time and I had to start removing my own personal weeds. The balance I created needed to be maintained, so that when I had to make more changes, it would be second nature. It took me three months at my new standard of smoking only twice a day. I constantly made the mistake of trying to bite off more than I could chew, and I always found myself slipping back into my old ways. That's why it's smart to balance yourself out before making major adjustments. I started focusing on making changes I could sustain instead of constantly getting ahead of myself.

Some people can consistently keep up with their new standard in a shorter amount of time. If you're disciplined and grow faster, go for it. Just make sure you can maintain that growth. I challenged myself to keep up with my new standard for ninety days before trying to grow beyond that point. As they say, it takes twenty-one days to create a habit, and I think ninety days starts to solidify whatever you're practicing.

When you feel like you have maintained proper balance over time, you've created a great foundation to begin a deeper detox. I want you to master balancing the scale and continue to maintain the new growth you've made. This builds confidence for when you really start to tip the scale away from smoking. It's a great platform before you begin to stretch yourself in uncomfortable but rewarding ways.

Chapter 5 Summary

1. In order to regain control, you want to start by building a strong foundation that helps you create the changes that you want.

2. Although redundant, to make any real changes you have to be sure to acknowledge your issue. Remember the hiker only knows his way by recognizing where he's at and where he wants to go, without it not much will happen.

3. Before beginning major changes start by just finding your halfway point. Don't try to quit or go days without smoking. Cut the number of times you smoke in a day in half and maintain that level for ninety days.

4. Balance is key to sustaining change.

5. It will be a complete lifestyle change, not a diet. Don't try to make major leaps. The point is for you to be able to maintain the new growth you've made.

CHAPTER 6:
MIRRORS

True progress in life comes from becoming an expert on yourself. You can create an environment and mindset to best suit your strengths and weaknesses by becoming fully aware of yourself.

My journey in changing my smoking patterns and habits came from me learning to be aware of my actions—internally and externally—so that I could change my patterns with the least amount of resistance. What I mean by *resistance* is anything that might tempt you to smoke or use cannabis, or anything that negatively impacts the growth you've made.

I focused on managing my emotions and surroundings when I was transitioning out of football. I was on the cusp of a major football contract, and I didn't know what direction it was going. I went to a rookie minicamp and was there for two weeks. My contract was on pause until I was to hear back from the coaches on whether I would play or not. I waited anxiously. That was all I had lined up for the year—and if it didn't work out, I wouldn't know what was next. The following week, the coaches told me they decided to go in a different direction. My contract to play was revoked and I had to figure out what was next.

After getting released, I had that feeling of being down, frustrated, and irritated. What do you think I did? I bought some weed and smoked it on the way home. I reverted to what had solved my issues for me in the past.

But that transition changed my smoking pattern so abruptly. As my great friend Gerald Howse often said, "Don't let your circumstances keep you from reaching your goals." At that time, I had no money coming in. The one and only thing I'd been doing my entire life, the career I thought was for me, had ended. I now had to make some changes and redirect my focus. Not knowing what I would do next dissolved my smoking habit rapidly. For the first time ever, I realized smoking wasn't going to help my problem. Smoking would only distract me from what was next and delay the inevitable. At that point I had to choose to face my problem and not run away from it.

I felt depressed sometimes if I didn't smoke. When I was frustrated, irritated, or aggravated—I impulsively chose to smoke. If I got high, I could relax. While I was trying to distance myself from weed, I went through a flood of emotions. I had good days, bad days, and days where I felt attached. The hardest days were when I tried to convince myself it was helping me. I was trying to center myself back to this balanced position of not letting it control me and dictate my happiness.

All of this took effort and caused me to develop in other areas I hadn't worked on before. I had to grow, which wasn't the most pleasant thing for me to do. Changing internally and externally wasn't comfortable, but it was necessary to keep me on track when I faced temptation. That's why I believe it's crucial to be aware of yourself, because it will be easier for you to adapt to change. Awareness is knowing yourself, knowing what best helps you cope, knowing your triggers, and knowing what makes you happy.

Develop External Awareness

While adapting, I began paying attention to external factors and eliminating anything that could cause resistance. I refer to this as *external awareness*, which helps when you're trying to create new patterns in your life. This means being aware of your environment or associations. A Japanese proverb states, "When the character of a man is not clear to you, look at his friends."

When I was younger, if you would have asked me if external factors can impact someone's life, I probably would have shaken my head in disagreement. I thought I could control anything and everything I did. If I wanted to do it, I would, and if I didn't, I wouldn't. I felt like I was good at controlling the choices I made even though I didn't always have the best people influencing me. I really followed only what I truly wanted to do.

I started to see the difference when I attempted to change some of the habits I didn't like in my life. It seemed like I couldn't catch any momentum. Every step forward led me to more resistance. The starting and stopping was irritating me, and I wondered what I was doing wrong.

I had a conversation with a close friend who told me about her process of changing. She explained how growing was difficult when she was involved with people who weren't on the same path. Not that it was bad, but it added resistance when she wasn't strong yet. For the moment, she had to remove herself from friends and family until she felt it was no longer an issue.

I started to understand where my struggles were coming from. I was continuing to be around the same group of friends who smoked weed multiple times a day, while trying to cut back myself. That wasn't working. By surrounding myself with them, I was creating more temptation. You already crave weed when you're trying to go without it, and I was making it harder by putting myself right in front of it.

When you're weaning off cannabis, allow yourself to gain some strength. For me, it was easier to not think about smoking when I was around people who didn't do it. My attention was somewhere else, and it was a great distraction. Soon I was strong enough to reject any temptation. Once I was aware of my environment, I was ready to work on my internal thoughts.

Create Internal Awareness

We all have internal battles that we have to overcome, and most of the time we ignore them. I had a lot of growing to do when changing my internal thoughts. Once I became aware of my surroundings, I had to learn to be internally aware.

I often convinced myself that I couldn't do something or that it was easier to give in. That conversation in my head always went against me, and I had to separate those thoughts from my actions. This made me start seeking good information to put into my head. I read books to help grow my mentality. I've never been a reader, but I needed to do things differently if I wanted to see a change.

If you think reading isn't for you, you can do other things to help yourself. For example, I often listen to podcasts, audio books, and practice meditating. All were helpful in maintaining a positive mental state. This helps you change how you process information and process things that happen to you.

In July 2019I spoke with Gloria Caldwell who has worked as a crisis counselor for over twenty-five years. She told me about internal awareness and how the application of information changes with each individual. She pointed out that our brain receives information in different ways. Each person processes information differently, and this affects how you perceive the information you're being given.

Think of the telephone game. One person whispers a message to the next, which is then passed onto the next person in line. By the time the message has reached the last person, it has completely changed from the original statement given. This game shows how people hear the same things but can perceive something totally different.

Internally, you have to carve out a place that's your safe haven in order to keep your thoughts on track. I never wanted to be an emotional hostage. So, when I hear the voice in my head telling me I need or want to smoke, I shift my focus—and this gets my thinking back on track.

Sometimes when we change our habits, our worst enemy is ourselves. The information we take in to help us can change, based on how we perceive and process things in our mind. That's why people with the same opportunity can end up with different results.

When you're trying to change your habit of smoking, remember to expand your mental capacity. Control your thoughts by feeding your mind positive information. Overall, you want to change the story you're telling yourself.

Always be aware of the negative thoughts roaming in your head—those thoughts telling you that you can't do something. The ability to catch these thoughts and replace them will help you respond to failures faster.

Recognition and Responsiveness

After practicing external and internal growth, practice quickly recognizing and responding to negative instances. I started to see a difference in how quickly I was able to catch negative thoughts or even take myself out of unhelpful environments.

I caught urges to smoke and redirected my focus or distracted myself. This continuous practice slowly took over. I remember a difficult week where I found myself smoking every day—but the following week I got back on track. I knew I slipped up, and instead of one week becoming one month of smoking, I caught myself.

In the beginning, it might take you longer to realize you're losing control. Practicing will help you shorten that length of time between each failure. It might not be pretty at first, but your recognition and responsiveness will become better.

Remember when you go through those internal and external battles, it will get easier to win. Creating a good environment for growth and building internal strength will help keep you strong and in control. It's one of the most important tools when learning to control the urge of using cannabis.

Chapter 6 Summary

1. Most addictions stem from other internal and external factors that you must be aware of before beginning to eliminate your dependency.

2. Get good at creating a healthy environment for yourself while adjusting your smoking habits. Surprisingly, who you choose to be around while growing can make it harder to change.

3. Start to overcome some of the internal battles that have led you to relying on weed.

4. The purpose of being aware of your thoughts and environment is to assist you in recognizing when you've gone off track, so you may alter your actions in order to find a better way.

CHAPTER 7:
PUSHING PATTERNS

Our daily patterns are a large indicator of our success. They either hurt or help us. Things we do easily become a part of our daily pattern. Something as simple as getting a coffee every morning from the Starbucks drive-thru can become habitual. We get to the point where we don't even think about it anymore, like brushing our teeth. It's no longer a question of whether you will or won't—because you've done it for so long, you don't even think about it anymore.

It's easy to be moved by the patterns you possess, yet some people overlook them and question why they may be in a certain situation. If you've ever wondered why you're where you're at with cannabis, the answer always leads back to your daily habits and patterns.

For example, I smoked for so long that people close to me knew my patterns of when, where, and what type of weed I was going to smoke. I was predictable to others and to myself, because the cycle I followed became something I naturally did with no thought. If you don't pay attention to your patterns, you can end up steering your future to a place you don't want to go. Take over the steering wheel and break the cycle that has become second nature.

Awareness is a key tool for gaining control of your daily cycles and triggers. Sometimes your triggers can dictate your patterns. Going back to the Starbucks example—why might someone grab a coffee at the drive-thru every morning? Most likely it's because they're tired and coffee gives them energy. The tiredness or lack of energy is the trigger to get a coffee.

When you're trying to quit or gain control, focus on making small changes to modify your triggers. I did this when I was changing my smoking habits. I realized I had reasons behind my smoking patterns. I was dealing with a range of emotions that prompted my smoking patterns. In order to get a different result, I needed to make adjustments.

Smoking Patterns and Daily Routine

When I consistently smoked, I had several patterns. My routine was solely based on emotional stress that I wasn't coping with. I used cannabis for increasing my appetite, physical wellness, and mental wellness. I would smoke before I ate, because for a period of time I had a poor appetite. I'm not sure why I wasn't hungry, but I knew that I could fix it by smoking. My solution was to plan my smoke sessions prior to eating. After getting into a routine of smoking before meals, I naturally created a habit. Smoking became an indicator of hunger. The end result was that I wouldn't eat unless I smoked before.

I also had a habit of smoking after practice and games to take the edge off. Really, I was using weed to self-medicate. Although doctors would prescribe opioids and other pain relievers, I didn't want to take those medications. As I mentioned before, I preferred cannabis, but as I used it to relieve my pain, it would also weave itself deeper into my life. I'm grateful I didn't get hooked on anything else. Nonetheless, I still created an unhealthy dependency.

For an attitude and personality boost, I liked to smoke before any functions, whether it was church, a day party, networking events, or family gatherings. The ones closer to me constantly questioned why I always had to smoke before anything I went to. Some pointed out how sociable I was when I was high. How I saw it was that I could relieve any nervousness and instead confidently interact at any type of event. I liked the fact that smoking made me calm, collected, funny, carefree, and positive.

Lastly, I got into the routine of smoking in high-stress situations. Whenever I was in circumstances that had a lot of stress or made me feel strong emotions, I smoked to calm myself down. I did this often, and I didn't develop great coping skills because of it. I used cannabis as an outlet instead of dealing with healthy alternatives to ease the emotions I was experiencing. This was one of the hardest hurdles for me to overcome, because it was much easier and less stressful to sweep my emotions under the rug instead of facing them.

Emotional and Physical Triggers

My patterns mostly came up due to underlying emotional and physical triggers. Many of the adjustments I made were modifying my emotions and physical pain. When you quit or try to gain control, you'll experience different triggers that are uncomfortable to handle without smoking. You have to remain strong and put strategies in place to deal with these. People have different triggers, so know which ones are yours, and be conscious of your patterns that follow them. Analyzing your routines will reveal most of your triggers, which is the starting point for creating a fitting solution.

My cravings to smoke were triggered by anxiety, insomnia, night sweats, lack of appetite, and uncontrollable emotions. These emotions were all super hard to face. It was even harder to face when

I had something like weed that could easily iron out the wrinkles.

Instead, acknowledge your triggers and solve them in a different way. There's usually an alternative way that solves the issue you want fixed. To illustrate, a lightbulb might be a good source of light, but a candle and the sun provide the same outcome that a lightbulb does, even though the amounts of light vary. Identify the cause of your smoking urges and choose to seek elsewhere for comfort, even when that level of comfort varies.

That being said, different triggers require different actions. I had to better myself in areas that were linked to my smoking patterns. The more direct and honest you can be with yourself about your struggle, the better. You want to be able to underline the reason behind the use, whether it's emotionally or physically relieving. When I was angry, sad, or anxious I just turned to smoking. Cannabis was my lifestyle. I found myself relying on weed to be the buffer between me and my issues. Choosing cannabis as a solution for a significant part of my life ended up creating a long list of triggers. I had to learn to change one thing at a time and start chopping at the roots of my habit.

This has been one of the most difficult concepts to master out of everything in the first quarter of life. My irresponsible use had some deeper meaning. I've said it before—I have a ton of regrets using all those years. But if my mistakes have helped me give insight to others, I'm glad to pay it forward.

Redirect Your Focus

Smoking was great because I wouldn't feel as overwhelmed by stressful situations. That's why I had to learn to smoke moderately and focus on handling stress in a better way. Moderation looks different for everyone. I know people who smoke only on the weekends, and I know people who set aside a few days a month to smoke. It's all about finding what works for you and making sure you're displaying habits that line up with what and where you want to be in the future.

The next step is to start redirecting your triggers. I started by switching up my routine and working on healthy ways to release a range of my emotions. It sounds simple, but it required effort and meant I had to keep myself busy. Sometimes it meant I had to have conversations and discuss my feelings with others to relieve some of the tension. I had to learn how to handle my feelings without using cannabis as a buffer.

Let's take my morning routine and dissect it so you have an example of redirecting your focus in a healthy way. As I said before, I had planned to smoke before most meals, which made it a part of my morning routine. A quick smoke session provided me with a good energy in the mornings. Anything after 1:00 p.m. would result in me feeling drowsy, unproductive, and hungry. I would smoke and eat a mango each morning before I started my day. I eventually made the adjustment of going for a run each morning instead of smoking. Running created natural dopamine, which gave me the energy and creativity I sought from smoking. By redirecting my attention, I stayed on the right track. When you're trying to reduce and change your habit, you need to have a positive replacement to fill the hole you've created. Referring back to my previous light analogy: same result, new source.

Keep in mind it can't just be any replacement— it has to be thoughtful and align with the need you seek to fulfill. For me exercise gave me a similar feeling of being "high" which worked perfectly to replace when I smoked. If the activity that your substituting doesn't align with that emotion that you seek from cannabis it likely will be short lived.

For a two-week streak, I attempted to take on guitar lessons as a replacement for smoking. I've always been fascinated with playing the guitar and I was sure it would be a great substitution to take my mind off smoking. After those two weeks, I dropped the ball. I may have liked the idea of playing the guitar, but I found the lessons extremely boring. Before I knew it, I went back to smoking before each lesson and it became a waste of time and money.

I continued my search for new sources of positive reinforcement. I went through several substitutions that ended up being unhelpful. They didn't fill the specific needs I was looking to fill, so I constantly went back to smoking. That's why it's a good idea to understand the triggers that follow your daily smoking patterns. From there, it's about finding similar activities to redirect your regular use of cannabis.

Chapter 7 Summary

1. Understanding your daily patterns and triggers can be a key component of gaining control of cannabis.

2. In some cases, most of our triggers are the cause of our habits. Be aware of triggers that may prompt you to use cannabis.

3. Be aware of any emotional and physical triggers that may cause you to want to use/ smoke cannabis.

4. Learn to redirect your focus in healthy ways that relieve stressors in the same way that cannabis has in past situations.

5. Remember that it can take time to find activities that give you the same relief that cannabis does. These activities need to con-sistently fulfill your needs.

CHAPTER 8:
THE PLAN

Having a plan is the number one thing I harp on. I can almost always connect a failure of mine to not constructing a plan. Prior to me achieving growth in this area, I wasn't much of a planner. I often led my life impulsively, and now I see that everything can go better when it's planned out beforehand. You don't have to be good at planning to get good at planning. It's a skill you can progressively get better at.

To improve planning skills, all you have to do is make your day a priority. Write down things you need to accomplish for yourself in order to not fall into using. Three things I focus on when planning are attainable objectives, active growth, and learned failures. Learning to plan and writing things down has been the reason for all my successes. If I wrote something out, it happened. The timeline I desired to accomplish my objectives may have varied, but nonetheless, I completed them. I like to think of writing things down as the power of suggestion. They say when you write something down, you're more likely to complete those tasks. Your mind finds solutions so that you can get where you want to go.

If you don't make a plan, you can become distracted from your vision. I convinced myself if I could keep busy, it would erase any chance for me to smoke. For example, I always made sure my schedule was full, in order to stay busy. Activities such as running, reading, playing video games, or attending social events—all helped divert my attention away from smoking. Make sure your activities are affiliated with places that don't tempt you to get high.

I wrote down productive learning areas I needed to improve, such as planning my week, meal prepping, and doing my daily meditation. As soon as I began filling my day with tasks, I started to think less about smoking. This took the focus off myself and how I felt, especially when I was craving weed.

Setting Objectives

Moving forward, you want to get really good at setting objectives and writing them down. This will help create thoughts that subconsciously work in your favor. For example, during my years playing football the team would take some time to meditate or visualize before the game. This helped direct the teams focus on what they wanted to achieve. Most of my thoughts were centered around plays I wanted to make or an overall mindset that I wanted to keep during the game. I really believe that visualizing those thoughts helped shift my mindset during the game.

That's why focusing and having tunnel vision helps keep you single minded on what you need to do. I like to think of it as being laser focused (precise and concise). All your objectives should be measurable, otherwise you're less likely to know if you're making progress. A measurable objective is saying, "I want to smoke once a day instead of twice a day." Measurable objectives are easy to analyze and monitor, which I'll explain in depth later in this chapter.

You also want to have attainable objectives, meaning objectives you can actually complete. Many people write down objectives that are too far of a stretch, then end up not seeing them through. Going slow and steady is acceptable when you're weaning off of cannabis, because it creates less cravings. Trying to quit cold turkey will only make you want it more.

My first objective was reducing the amount of times I smoked down to once a week. This was too much of a stretch because previously I'd been smoking every day. After a month of missing the mark, I doubted my ability to control my habit at all. Setting my objective out of my reach crushed my confidence. I struggled to gain progressive momentum. The lack of progress caused me to adjust my strategy and learn how to set objectives for growth versus speed. That's when I started setting objectives that were more doable and less challenging.

So, what objectives should you make? Think about how much you smoke, why you smoke, and when you smoke. Where you're at in these areas should determine what objectives you set. Maybe your objectives overlap with personal growth aside from your cannabis consumption. One of my objectives was to get good at addressing my emotions, so I set a goal to talk to someone once a week about my feelings instead of denying them every time I felt upset. Although it wasn't directly focused on weed, it was still linked to why I wanted to smoke.

After you've determined your objectives and written them down, write different activities to replace the times when you would normally consume. Keep these activities in mind when you're trying to find a solution for your smoking habit. These activities should be unique to you and based on your interests. I found it helpful to have several ideas to distract me from smoking when I normally would.

Try to focus on maintaining your garden and balancing out your smoking habits. After thinking about objectives, you're ready to write them down. I preferred writing my objectives in a journal and my schedule of activities in a planner. Every Sunday I took about forty-five minutes to an hour to write all of my objectives and scheduling activities for the week. All the objectives I had were paired with those activities in place of when I would normally smoke. For instance, when my objective was to smoke every other morning, I scheduled my runs or my activity for the same day and time.

I found reading, family gatherings, and friend outings to be helpful for taking my mind off smoking. This may not be the right fit for you, so get creative and take the time to find out what works for you. I tested many things before I found out what activities would work. I liked outdoor activities, such as hiking. During the weekends when I had more time on my hands, I found hiking to be helpful because it was challenging and time-consuming.

Active Growth and Tracking

Once you find good activities as substitutions for your normal routine, start looking back at those objectives for the week. Put them somewhere you can see them—that way, you can always read them. Now it's time to take action and work toward decreasing the number of times you smoke or use cannabis. As you conquer your objectives, you'll continue to make new objectives until you've taken total control of your dependency. This is the active growth portion of your plan. Active growth is taking steps forward to get you where you want to be. If you're not taking action and following through with objectives you set, you won't move forward in gaining control.

I found it helpful to see the progress I was making instead of guessing if I was making any progress. We often convince ourselves we're making tons of progress when we actually aren't. Your plan should be accompanied by tracking, because it helps you get an idea of where you need to challenge yourself and where you may need to adjust. Each week I tracked, I gained insight on what I could improve on for the next week. Tracking can be tedious, but it adds so much value when you're forming new habits.

When you're tracking your objectives, keep it as simple as possible. Set one to two weekly objectives, then see which daily steps you need to take to be successful. I say weekly instead of monthly because sometimes looking too far ahead can be distracting and discouraging to your daily progress. Focus on one day at a time versus thinking about longer periods of time.

Failure Is Good

As you're tracking and initiating your plan to cut back on smoking or using cannabis, remember that you'll face failure. The whole reason I wrote this book was to show how much and how often I've failed. My hope is that I can give you advice to lessen the amount of times you fail, but just know that failing is a part of success. Failure comes with change and learning, and without it, we would never get better. It's similar to a baby learning to walk for the first time. The only way they improve is by falling and getting back up over and over again. If a toddler decided to give up after they fell once, they would never learn to walk.

You have to view failure differently than it's normally taught. Most failure is accompanied with a sense of loss or shame, but that's not how we should view it. You're learning and changing lifestyle patterns. Failure is only bad if you keep making the same mistake and aren't progressively learning from it. So fail over and over again, with one twist though: evaluate each failed attempt so that you learn from each experience. If you repeatedly make the same mistakes without making adjustments, you won't make any progress.

Prolonged thinking allows our brain to find a solution to any problem. However, most people don't take the time to think through their failures. This makes it more likely for them to face the same failure numerous times. As you meet your failure, take the time to make adjustments so that you progressively grow. That doesn't mean you won't run into a brick wall every once in a while. I've found myself running into the same mistake numerous times before figuring out a solution. Sometimes it takes more than one evaluation to find out the best way to prevent you from missing your mark.

Chapter 8 Summary

1. Having a plan is important because it lets you know the steps that you want and need to focus on in order to grow.

2. When making a plan, write out your objectives. What things do you intend to change in order to gain control? Start with three objectives and add on to them as you complete each objective.

3. Objectives should be measurable so that you can monitor and analyze your progress.

4. Don't set objectives that are too far of a stretch, it ends up hurting your confidence rather than helping it.

5. After you have found good substitutions that will replace your normal patterns, you want to begin actively living out your plan.

6. Evaluated failure is necessary for growing. Always make sure you understand that evaluating your failures is how you get better and get closer to controlling your habit.

CHAPTER 9:
LIVE FREE

We all have something we struggle with in the area of self-control. (For my friend, it's bread. She loves bread. It's nonstop. She'll do two workouts in a day, then go eat some bread. I don't get it.) For me, it was smoking weed. For you, it might be something else. Whatever your habit is, the goal is to gain self-control, which brings freedom.

It took me many years to get to a place where I felt free from cannabis. So just know that reaching your freedom may take time. The goal is to chip away at your habit a little bit at a time. If you do a little work every day, you'll get where you want to be. It's just a matter of time. The only way you'll fail is if you quit and don't follow through with your plan.

Continue to look over the things that have helped you through trial and error. By doing this you will relieve yourself from making the same mistakes that you have made in the past. The errors that have presented themselves throughout your journey will become great indicators of growth. This will be apparent, as long as you're reflecting on these instances. Pay attention to when and where you see the most improvement.

I started redirecting my smoking routine in 2015. From there it took consistent effort just so I wouldn't take steps backward. Every time I deviated from my plan of action, I found myself working twice as hard to get back on track. There were times when I had to start all over and devise a new plan because reflecting on my failures would change the direction that my plan needed to go. I always thought of this process like Google Maps or any other form of GPS. When there's an accident or maybe construction, it will recognize those delays and find an alternate route that will get you to your destination faster. The tools I've given you are same things I had to revisit and work on countless times until I felt in control. The idea is that whatever you've found to replace cannabis will become your new way of living.

Revisit Your Why

Creating a healthy lifestyle is a long-term process. Even after you've gained control, you can still be tempted and slip up. That's why I continue to revisit the objectives I had in my plan and know that you might have to regularly. Revisiting all the struggles I faced was an excellent tool to help me maneuver around my weaknesses. If your end objective is seeking a more permanent change, then you will always have to keep working on implementing healthy habits. Changing the role cannabis has played in your life isn't meant to be temporary, so don't treat it like a fad diet.

I grew and found myself strong enough to withstand any temptation, but that wasn't always the case. There were days I didn't feel as strong and continued to follow the principles I practiced before I could stay on track. Let's face it—cannabis isn't going anywhere any time soon. So, remind yourself of the work you did. Moments that test you make you stronger and help solidify your new habits. It's similar to that brief moment before you begin your work out. Not many people enjoy it, but after you complete it, you feel much better and even a sense accomplishment.

You'll get to a point where you start to look at cannabis differently. The times of revisiting will decrease, and one day it'll be like brushing your teeth. You won't think about whether you'll fall back into your old smoking patterns because you've created a new norm.

Living Above It

A friend once told me we never get rid of our demons; we just learn to live above them. I've always needed freedom in all areas of my life. I never wanted to be controlled by any of my weaknesses. That's why I needed to grow and stop letting cannabis be the lead role in my life.

I remember the day I wrote out my objectives and created a plan to change my smoking patterns. It was my sophomore year in college. I had a sticky note that said, "You won't reach what's in front of you, if you're not willing to let go of what's holding you back." I'm not sure who said that, but I posted that sticky note on the wall by the side of my bed so that I had a constant reminder of the person I was fighting to be. All the years of looking at that message pushed me to keep going until smoking was no longer at the center of my life.

After seeing that sticky note for three years, I finally took it down. I glanced at the wall and recognized the note had served its purpose. I reached over and crumbled it up, knowing it was the last time I would let weed control me. I finally felt like the childhood Tarris again—full of life, aspirations, and curiosity. I restored my love for doing things without being high. It was tough at times, especially when I was around friends who still smoked, but I developed confidence from years of learning and growing.

I was done rolling my problems into blunts. I was looking forward to conquering whatever was next. The next step for me was to help others become free from their dependency. Witnessing my shake back was great, but I wanted to help others realize they can free themselves from their dependency if they tailor their life to make them more of a controlled smoker.

Playing to Win

As I was putting this book together, I got an opportunity to speak with the McEachern High School football team about smoking cannabis. I had randomly bumped into their head coach and in our conversation the topic of my book came up. The head coach discussed how some of the players smell like weed all the time. After telling him about the struggles I've gone through he insisted that I give his team some insight on smoking weed. Their team was known for producing greats, and he felt like I would be able to reach some of the athletes in a positive way. Of course, I agreed and proceeded to set up a date and time to go speak with the team.

I won't lie I felt weird that I would be telling a group of young kings what they should or shouldn't be doing. I wasn't sure if I would even reach any of them, knowing that a younger me would be reluctant to listening. I shared some of the battles I went through and the things I've learned from smoking for all those years.

At the end of my speech, I warned the young players, "Smoke it, but don't let it smoke you." The team clapped. Then they made their way out of the room. After speaking with the coach, I went to the locker room to use the restroom before hitting the road. As I walked in, I smelled the familiar aroma of cannabis coming from one of the stalls. I figured the boys were rolling up and weren't aware I was present. As I came closer to the stalls, I overheard one boy say, "Man, just make sure you don't let it smoke you." I proudly grinned to myself, knowing that one boy understood the message I wanted them to take away.

One conversation with a high-school football team reached someone who changed his own perspective and influenced others. That boy is why I speak and why I chose to write this book. I hope it inspires others to create awareness and share their own story, because I can only relate to so many people.

Realize that your story is powerful and can help others too. The value of sharing struggles goes beyond what we see. I didn't even know the young man's name, but my message reached him. I hope he continues to pass that message on to others.

That's how change begins—the choice to speak up and be vulnerable with others, so that they can learn and do better.

Chapter 9 Summary

1. When you gain self-control over cannabis you will always need to make sure you revisit why you wanted more control in the first place. This helps sustain the changes that you have made.

2. There will be days that are harder than others and it will be tempting to go back to old ways, just remind yourself of the work you did and know that hard moments help build you even stronger.

3. You will get to a point where you look at weed in a different way and it's not something that you depend on anymore, and it will be the biggest relief to know that you control your life's progress, not weed.

4. Be the best version of yourself and help others through the growth and failures that you have experienced. Passing on what we have conquered is more powerful and more fulfilling than you know.

CHAPTER 10: CONCLUSION

Writing this book was like therapy for me. It helped me to stop getting in my own way and to live the lifestyle I've always wanted to live. It let me conquer my fear of not maximizing my potential in all areas of my life. I always wanted to live a fulfilled life where I can buy gifts for my family and friends, be a great dad and husband, be a great example, and handle tough situations well. I've always wanted to do what I want to do, when I want to do it. But with the amount I smoked, the money I spent, the time I wasted, and the emotions I blocked, cannabis wasn't getting me where I wanted to go.

I never thought I'd write a book about how to control the role cannabis played in my life to help others. My close friends and family jokingly refer to me as "the weed guru" because of all the trips I've taken and research I've done for this book. Now more than ever, I have cannabis all around me. I live in a state where it's legalized and, as I said before, I have several dispensaries within a mile from my place. Luckily, I've gained enough self-control so that I'm not constantly getting high off the endless supply that surrounds me.

People ask me all the time if I think cannabis is bad or if I would do things differently, knowing what I know now. Because cannabis doesn't show harmful side effects right away like other drugs do, it's easy to misuse it and justify your behavior. The side effects creep up on you and before you know it, cannabis has woven itself into your life and become a part of who you are rather than what you do. For that reason, I think cannabis is conducive to addiction.

I also recognize it's one of the healthier drugs out there in relation to effects they have on the mind and body. I'm not against it, but I'm not suggesting you should take using it lightly.

Now that the legalization movement has begun to spread, it's commercialized and advertised more than ever. Availability has sparked easier access to the drug, so I expect people's use will ramp up even more. If you use it, don't let it dictate your daily decisions. Don't let it control you. Find the balance, and don't become dependent on cannabis to remove the responsibility you have to yourself.

If I was given the chance to go back and do things differently, I could proudly say I wouldn't. The fact is that my struggles with weed have paved a way for me to help others, and I love that. I can now add value to others based on the failures I've lived. To me, that's the greatest thing that has come from my struggles.

I hope my story has inspired you to gain control over your habit so that you can excel in areas that truly matter to you. Let my story shatter any limitations you—or anyone else—has put on you. Find the courage to step outside of your comfort zone and develop the greatness within you. Free yourself so that your garden can grow far beyond what you thought it ever could.

And remember—if you choose to smoke weed, don't let it smoke you.

AFTERWORD

If you found value in this book, please pass it on to other people you know who might be in similar situations. If you don't want to go on this journey alone, I have a program where I will personally walk you through the plan I created for myself. It will assist you and help you dissect your specific situation so that you're successful in your growing process. For information on this program, email me at dontletitsmokeyou@gmail.com.

For more of my stories, tips, struggles, and thoughts on cannabis and finding balance, check out my blog, Clever Chief (www.cleverchief.org). I'd love to hear from you about your own relationship with cannabis and how you grew to become better.

NOTES

1. Eli McVey, "Chart: Recreational marijuana stores are clustered in low-income areas of Denver, Seattle," *Marijuna Business Daily*, July 31, 2017, https://mjbizdaily.com/chart-recreational-marijuana-stores-clustered-low-income-areas-denver-seattle/.

2. "The History of Medicinal Cannabis," Montana State Legislature, August 2010, https://leg.mt.gov/content/Committees/Interim/2009_2010/Children_Family/Emerging-Issue/mmga-presentation-cannabis-history-aug2010.pdf.

3. Stephen Siff, "The Illegalization of Marijuana: A Brief History," *Origins* 7, no. 8 (May 2014): https://origins.osu.edu/article/illegalization-marijuana-brief-history.

4. Peter Guither, "Why is Marijuana Illegal?" Drug Warrant, http://www.drugwarrant.com/articles/why-is-marijuana-illegal/.

About the Author

Tarris Batiste had a complicated relationship with weed starting in middle school. As a child, he developed a smoking habit and saw firsthand how damaging it is to lack self-control. While playing football at Georgia State University, he was drafted by the Atlanta Falcons, but life had different plans for him.

Today Tarris coaches people to get control of their dependency, using the motto "Smoke it—but don't let it smoke you." He helped start a nonprofit called the"Circle of Advancement, which gives students in northern Georgia guidance on life after high school or college. He has an MBA. For more information, visit www.cleverchief.org.